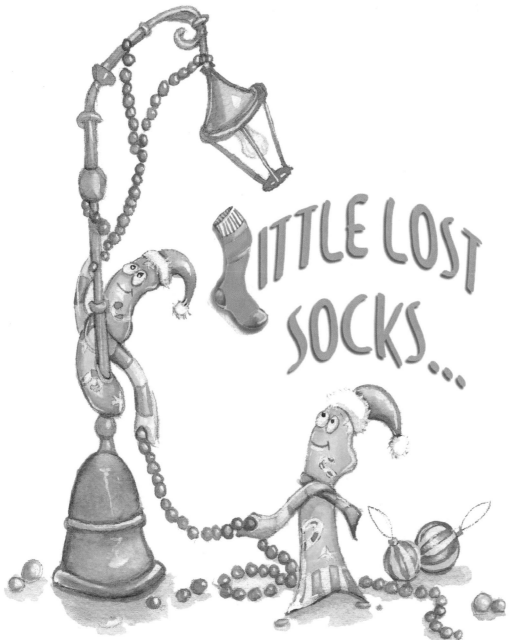

# LITTLE LOST SOCKS...

## BY DEEANN SCHUMACHER
## ILLUSTRATED BY
## EMMA STUART

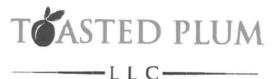

ISBN: 978-1-7329334-1-5

This book is a work of fiction. Places, events, and situations in this book
are purely fictional and any resemblance to actual persons, living or dead,
is coincidental.

Dedication DeeAnn Schumacher
This book is dedicated to Jesus Christ our lord
and savior. He turns "scars into stars" for the
glory of his holy name. The most beautiful three
little words in the world were spoken by Jesus
when he said "it is finished." What looked like a
failure through worldly eyes was a success, a
victory in God's eyes. He has given us the last
page first. Choose the winning side. Choose Jesus.

Dedication Emma Stuart
I dedicate this book to my little boy
Redmond Stuart Betheras who I snuggle
and read to every night...

# LITTLE LOST SOCKS...

Pendrell sat up
and looked around,
wondering where he
was and how he got there.

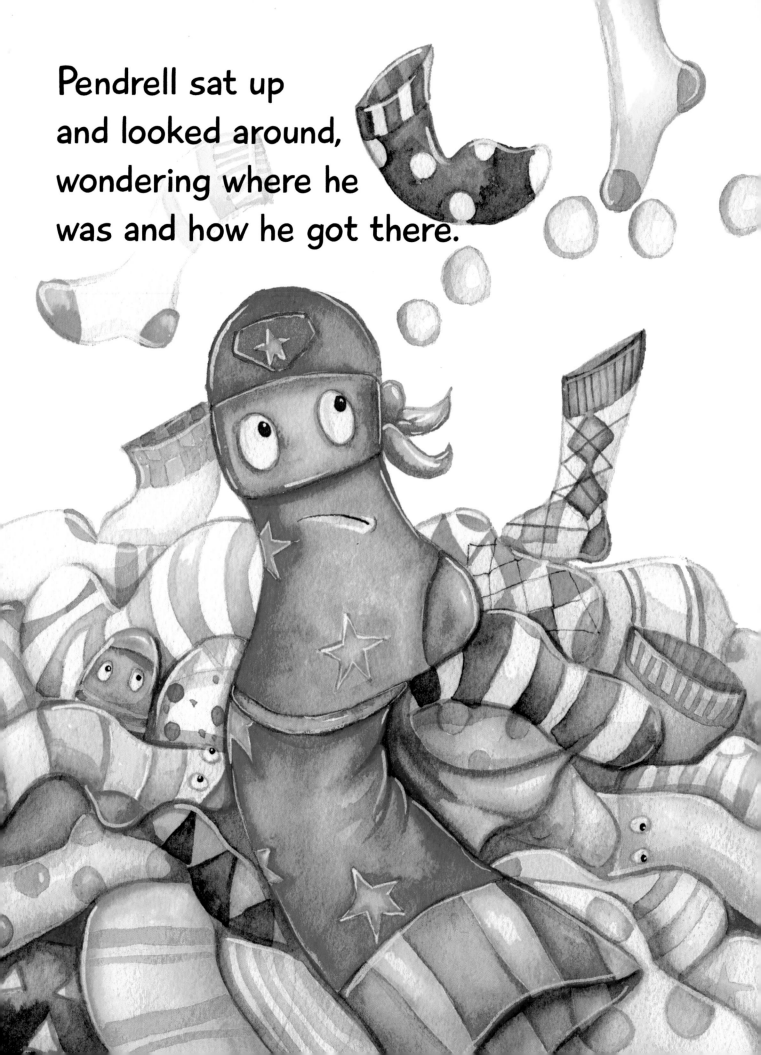

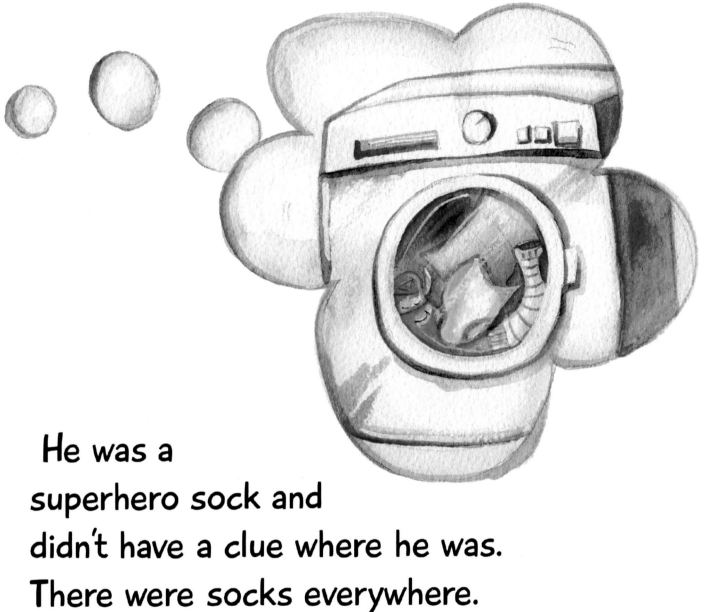

He was a
superhero sock and
didn't have a clue where he was.
There were socks everywhere.
Socks he had never seen before or
shared a drawer with. The last thing he
remembered was tumbling through the dryer.

A pink lace ankle sock appeared out of thin air, right before his eyes.

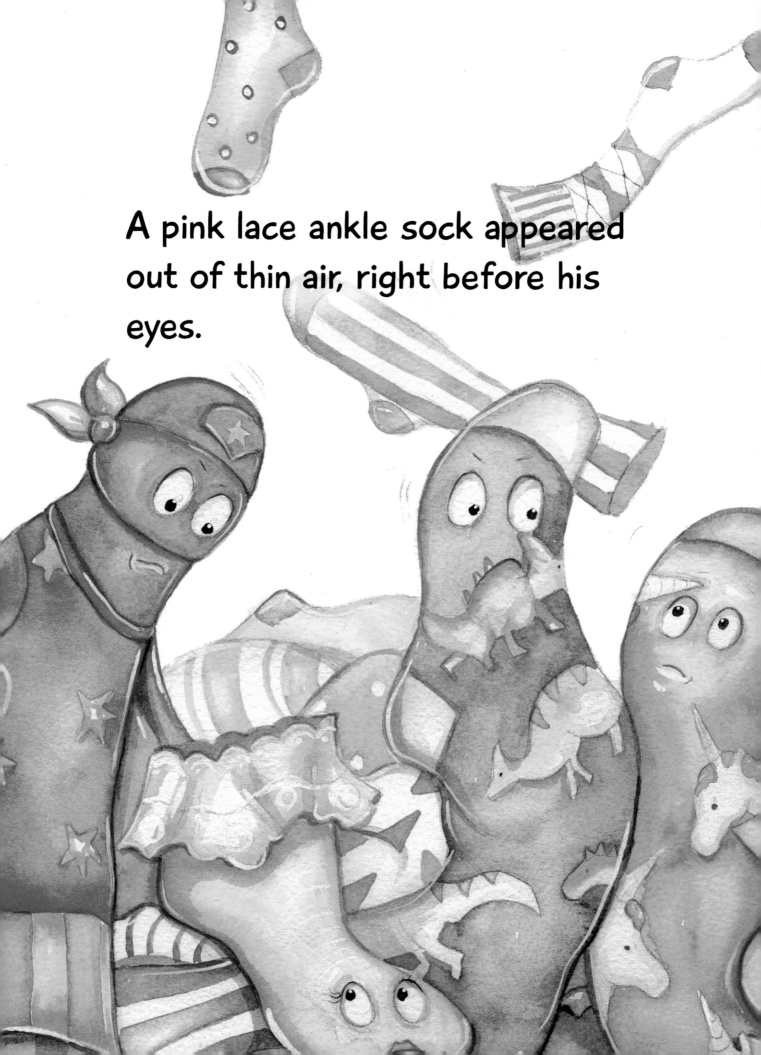

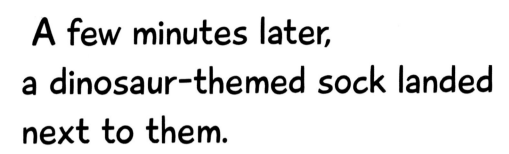

A few minutes later,
a dinosaur-themed sock landed
next to them.
Then, a sock decorated with
unicorns joined the group.

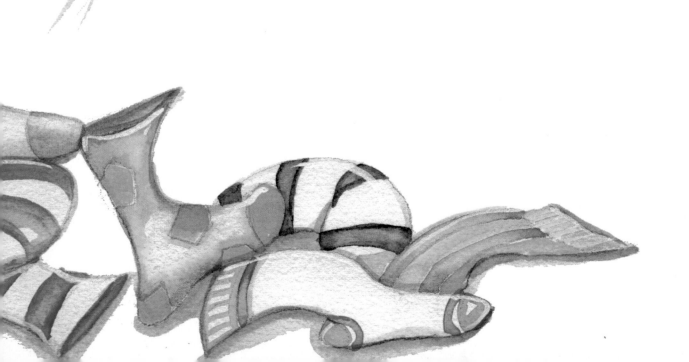

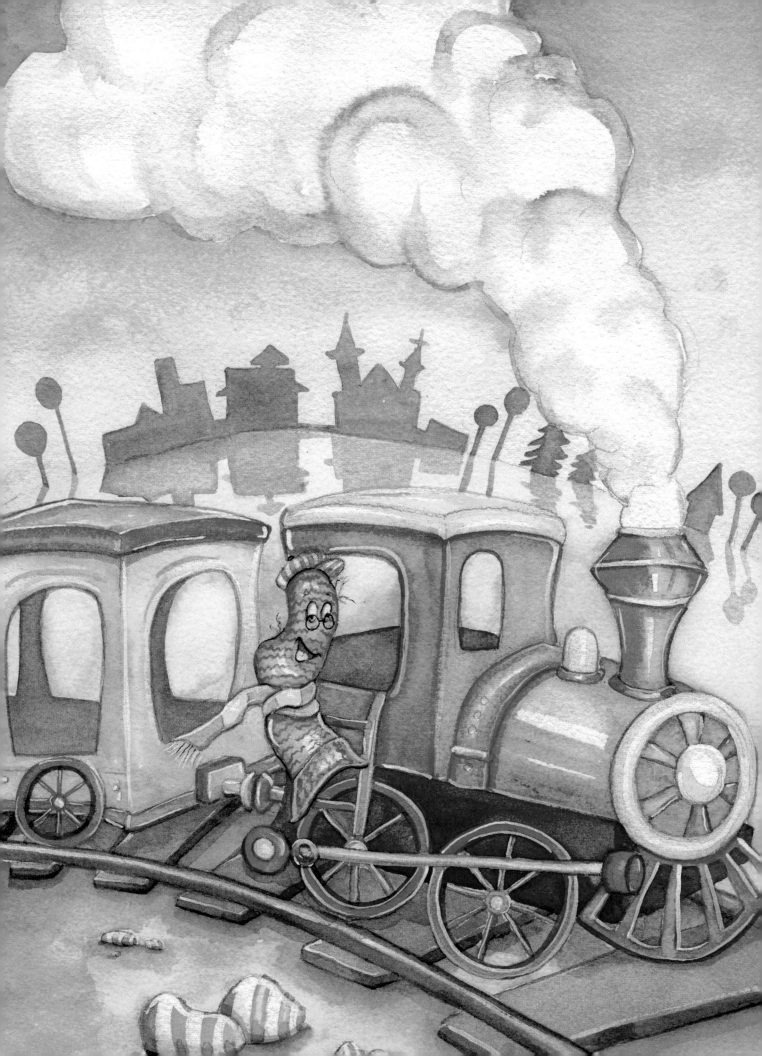

They were all confused but not afraid.
Somehow, they had just been dropped
into a colorful fairytale. A tall wool
sock stepped off the train that just
pulled up and greeted them.
He welcomed them to the Land of the
 Lost Socks.

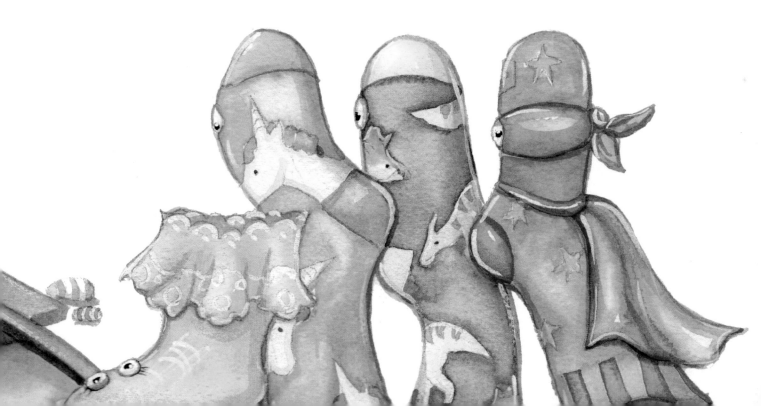

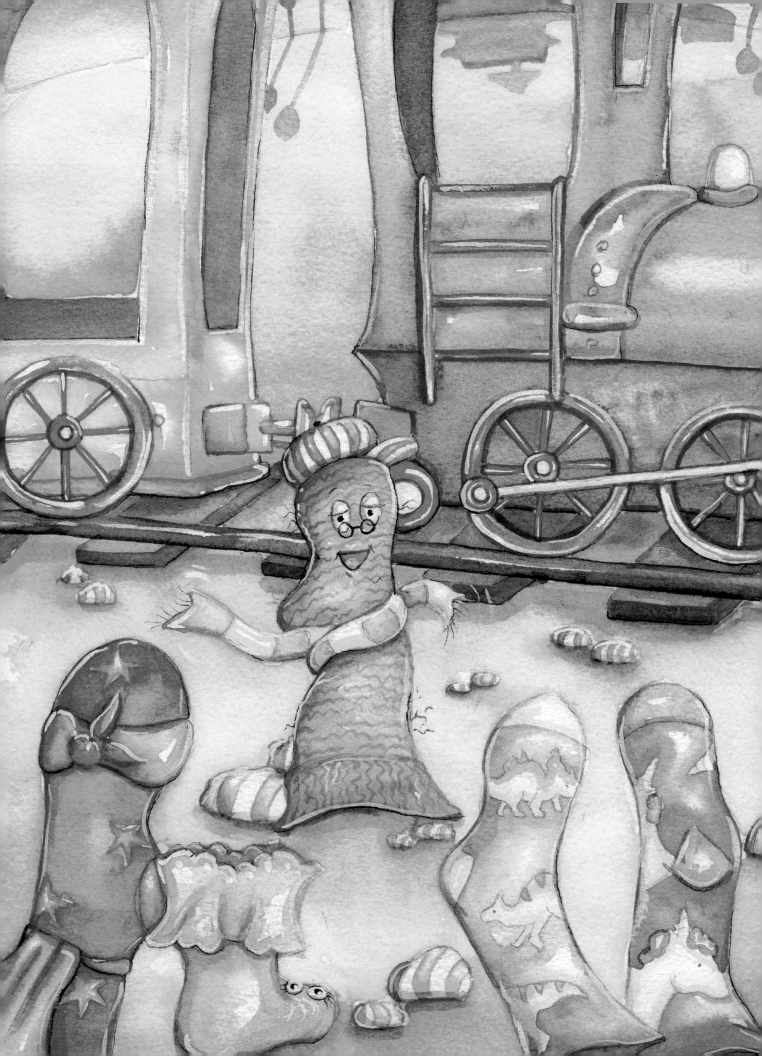

Wool Sock explained to
  them that this is the place
where all lost socks end up
when they have lost their soulmate.
It's a home and safe haven for
  mismatched socks.
The mystery is not fully
understood, but socks get
  pulled into a special gateway
and free-fall into this world.
They return home in the opposite
direction if they choose to go
  back and be found.

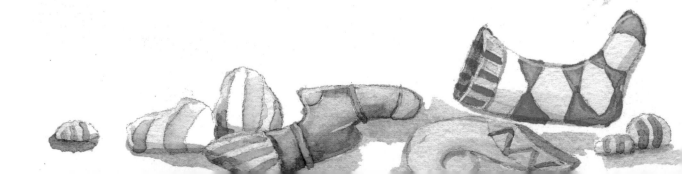

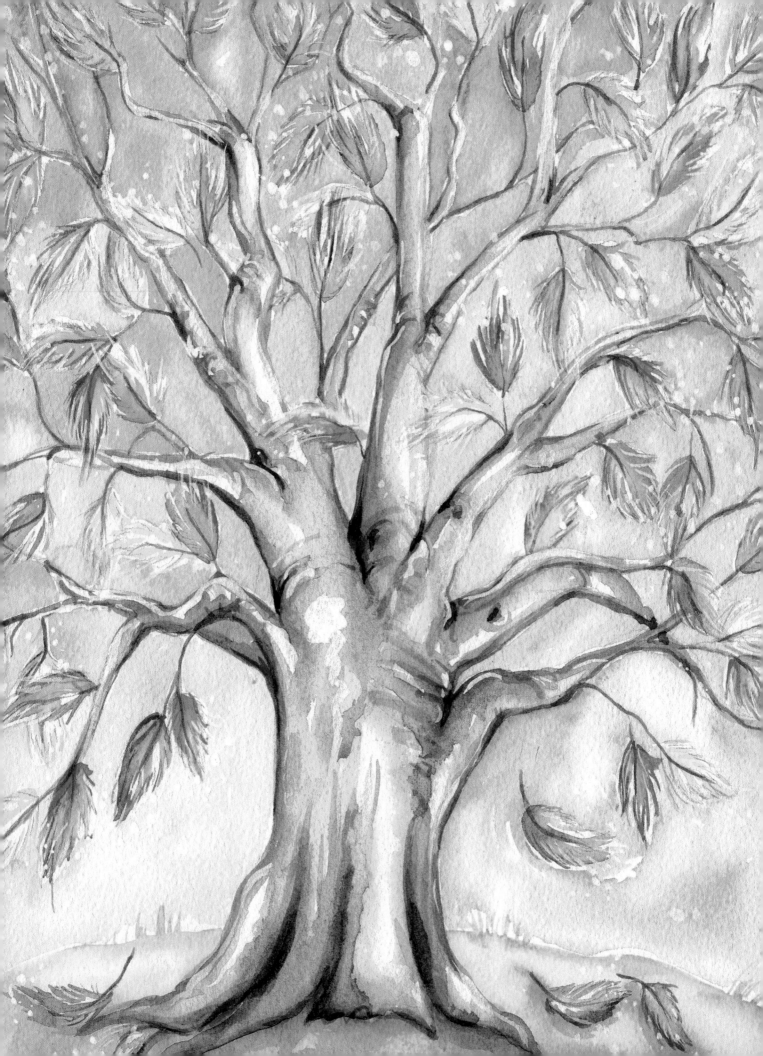

All new arrivals are given a train ride through town to get acquainted before they make their decision. At the end of the guided tour is a wishing tree where the new socks will be prompted to make a wish to stay or leave.
It is entirely their choice.

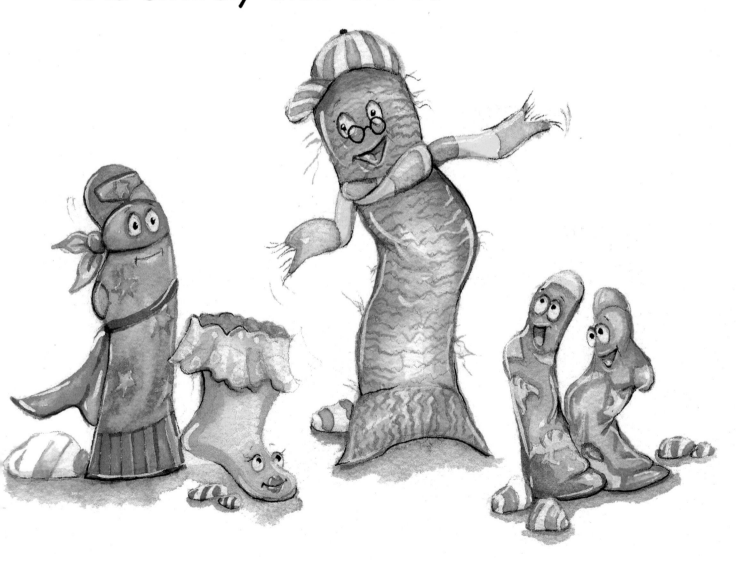

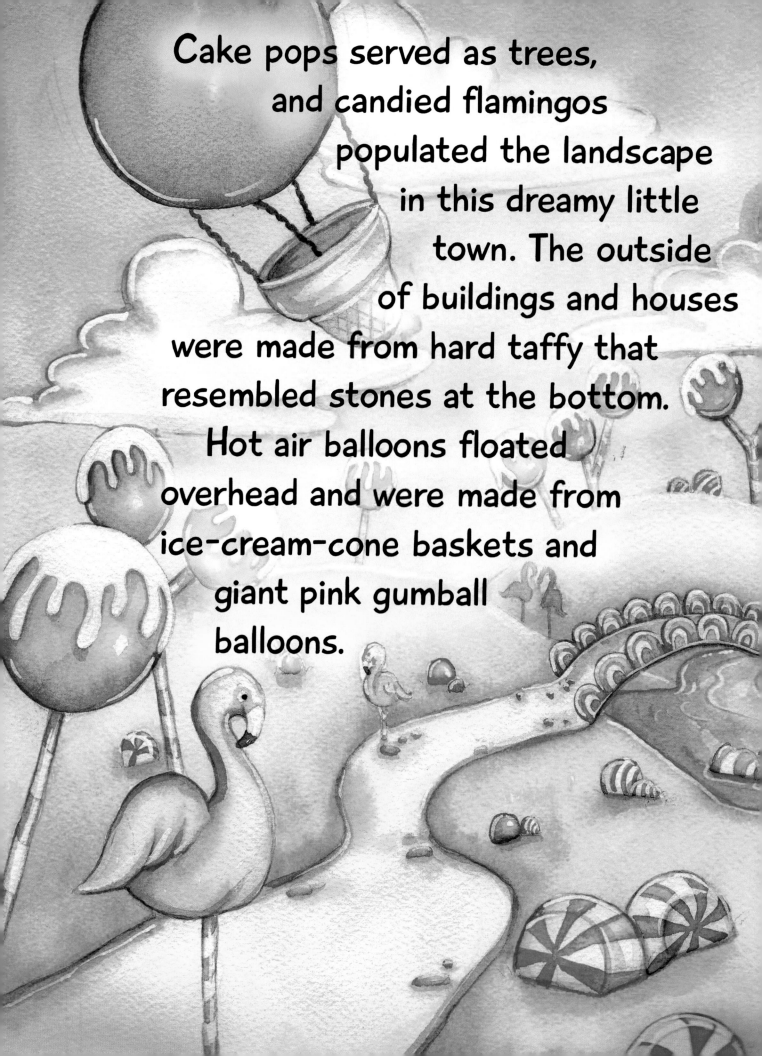

Cake pops served as trees, and candied flamingos populated the landscape in this dreamy little town. The outside of buildings and houses were made from hard taffy that resembled stones at the bottom. Hot air balloons floated overhead and were made from ice-cream-cone baskets and giant pink gumball balloons.

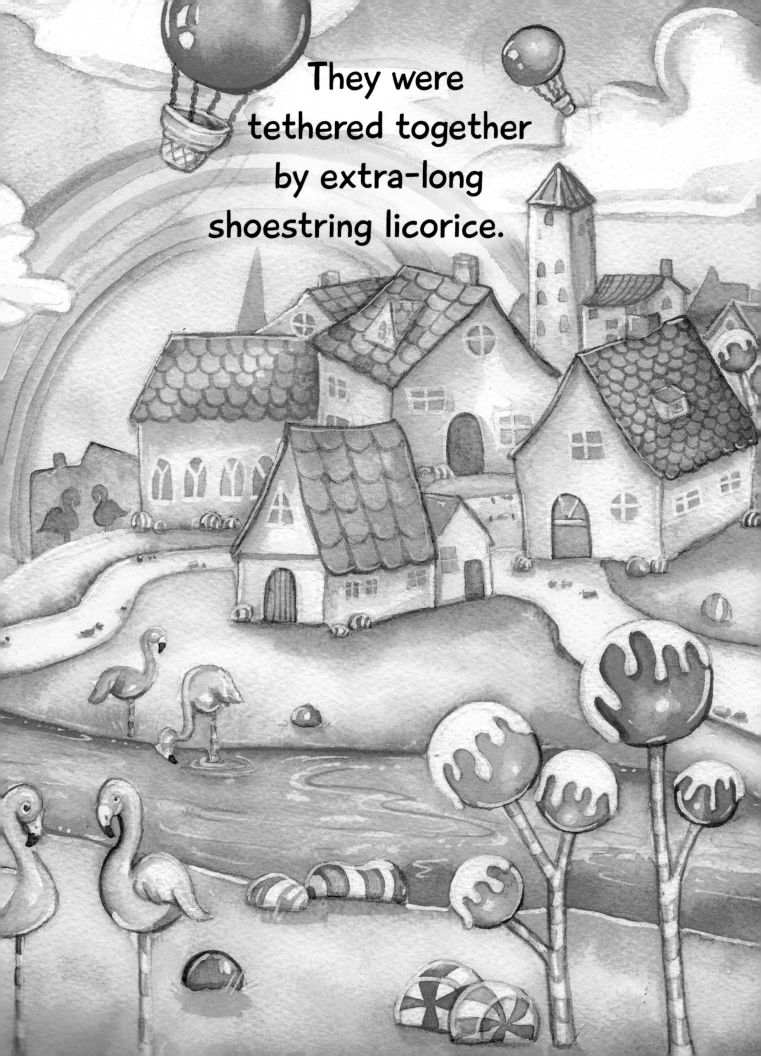

They were
tethered together
by extra-long
shoestring licorice.

Wool Sock was a weathered old sock, the oldest in fact, and the wisest sock around. He served as the train conductor, tour guide, and mentor.

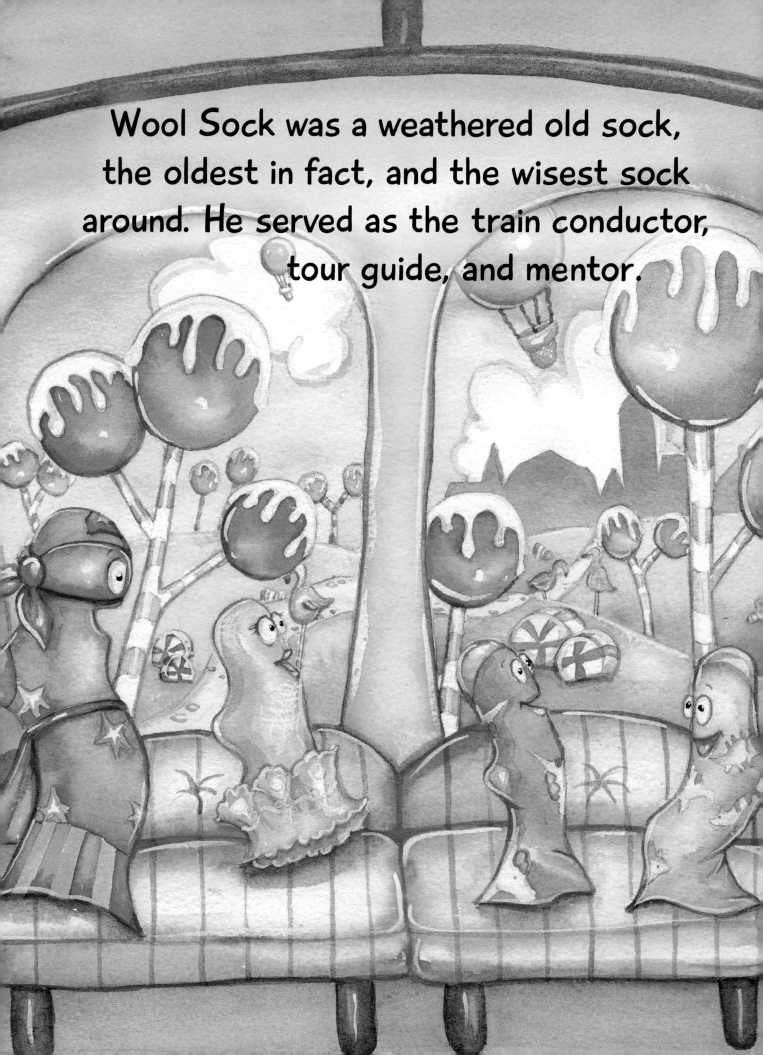

He still remembers
what it was like to be
the new sock in town
and how anxious he
was upon arrival.
Change is never easy,
especially when it happens so unexpectedly.
Wool Sock's goal was to help new socks
find a common interest in each other
to help them make friends easier.

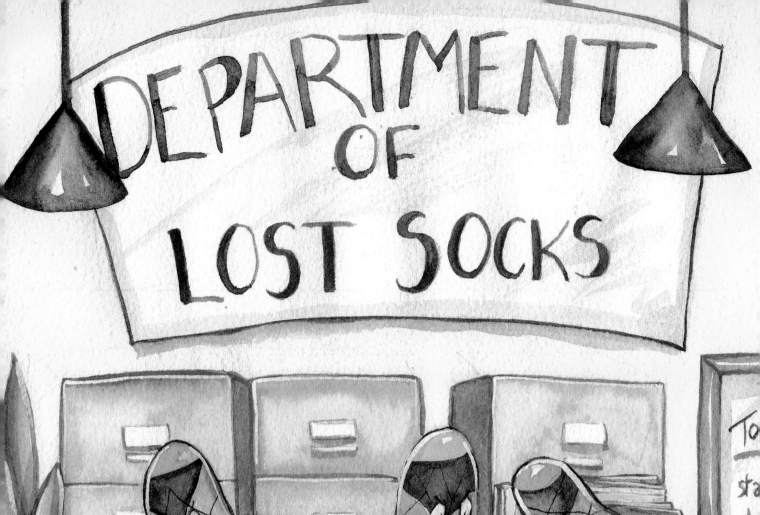
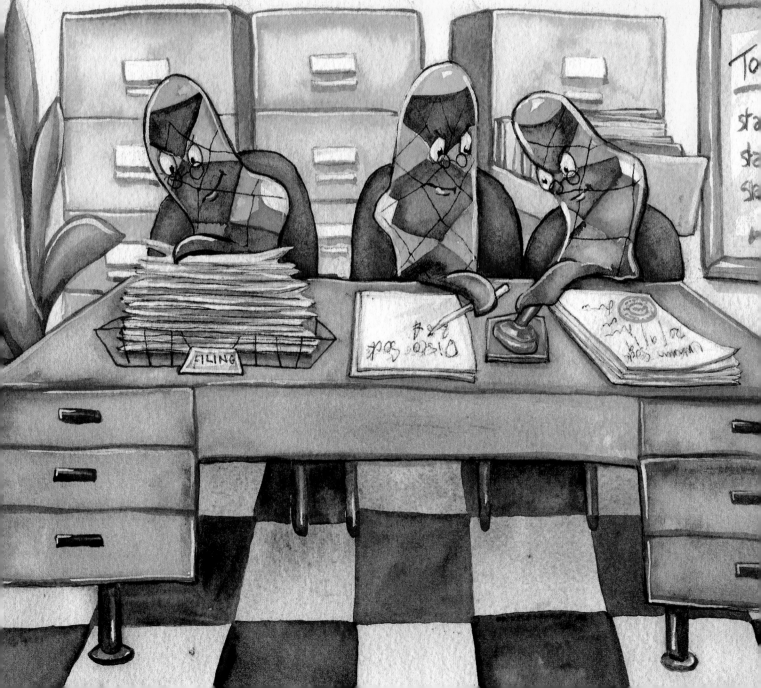

Wool Sock instructed the socks to climb aboard then blew the whistle as the train pressed its way to the checkpoint. The Department of Lost Socks was the first stop.

Every new sock had its name, date of arrival, and other important information written in a record book. The argyle dress socks usually worked the office jobs and handled this task. They kept meticulous records about each sock.

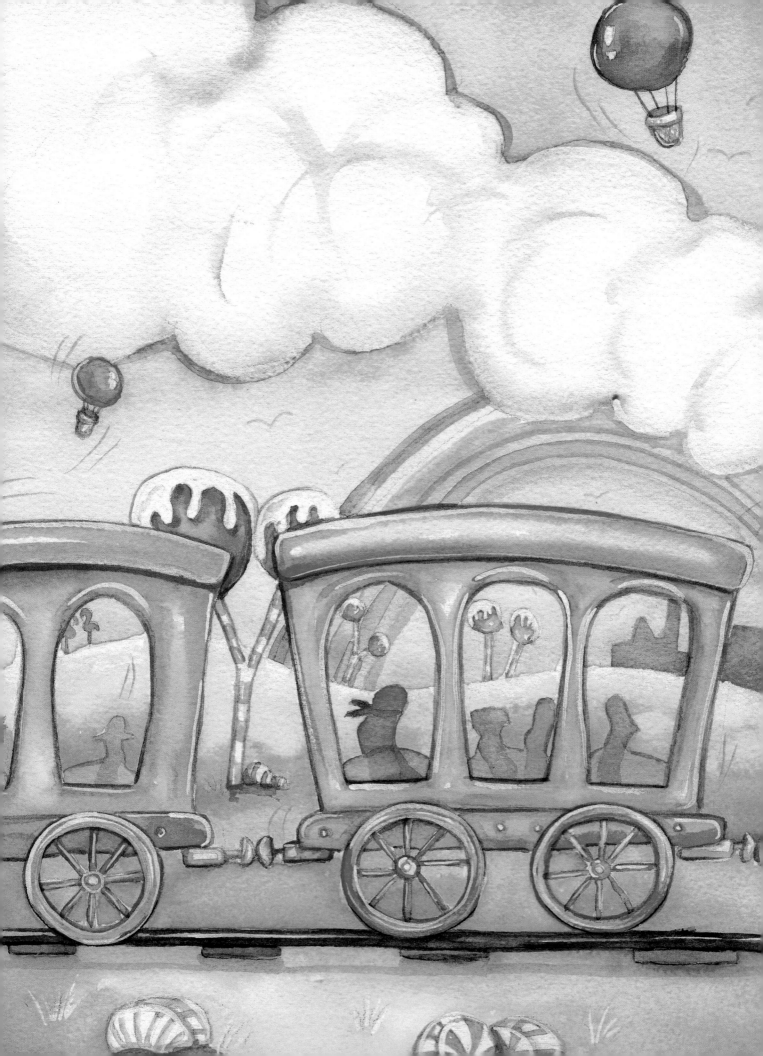

Wool Sock started the day by having the socks introduce themselves before they got checked in. Afterward, he called out to the new passengers to climb aboard once again.
The whistle blew,
the train snorted,
and the wheels rolled.

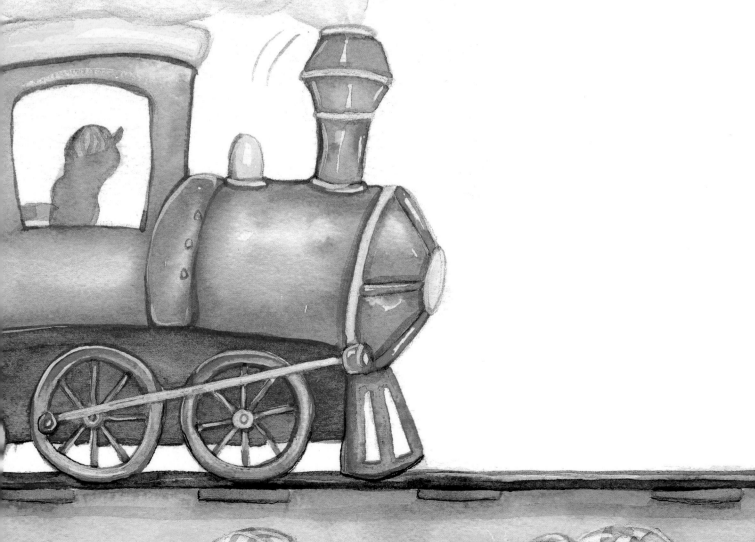

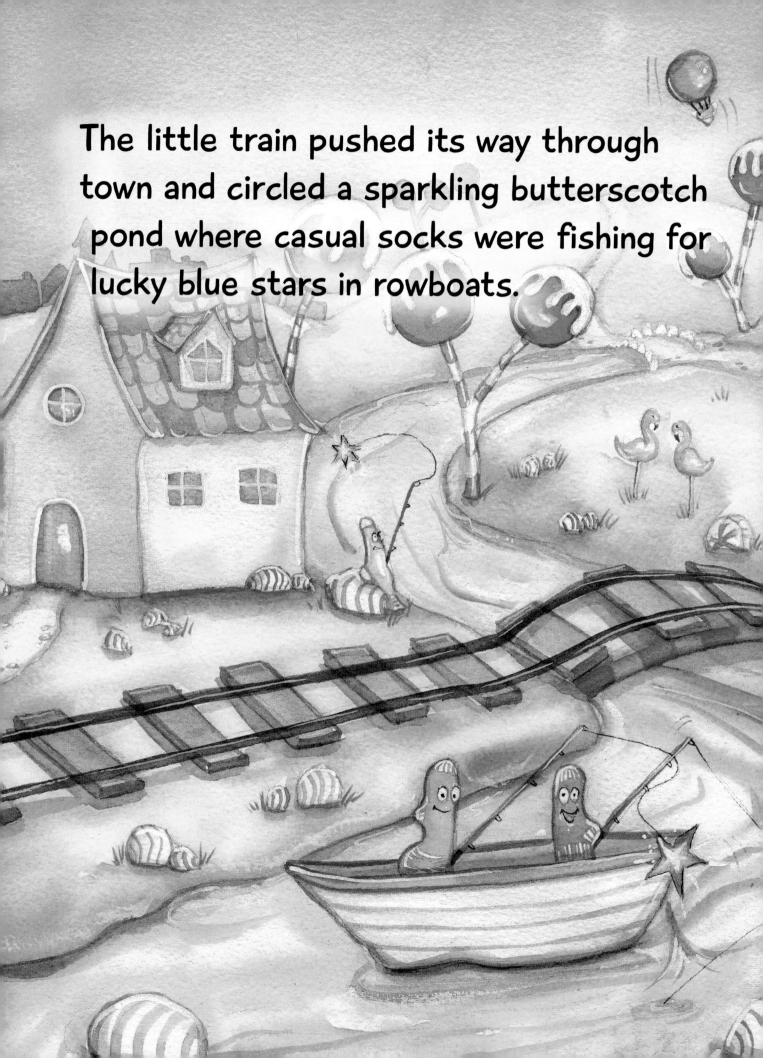

The little train pushed its way through town and circled a sparkling butterscotch pond where casual socks were fishing for lucky blue stars in rowboats.

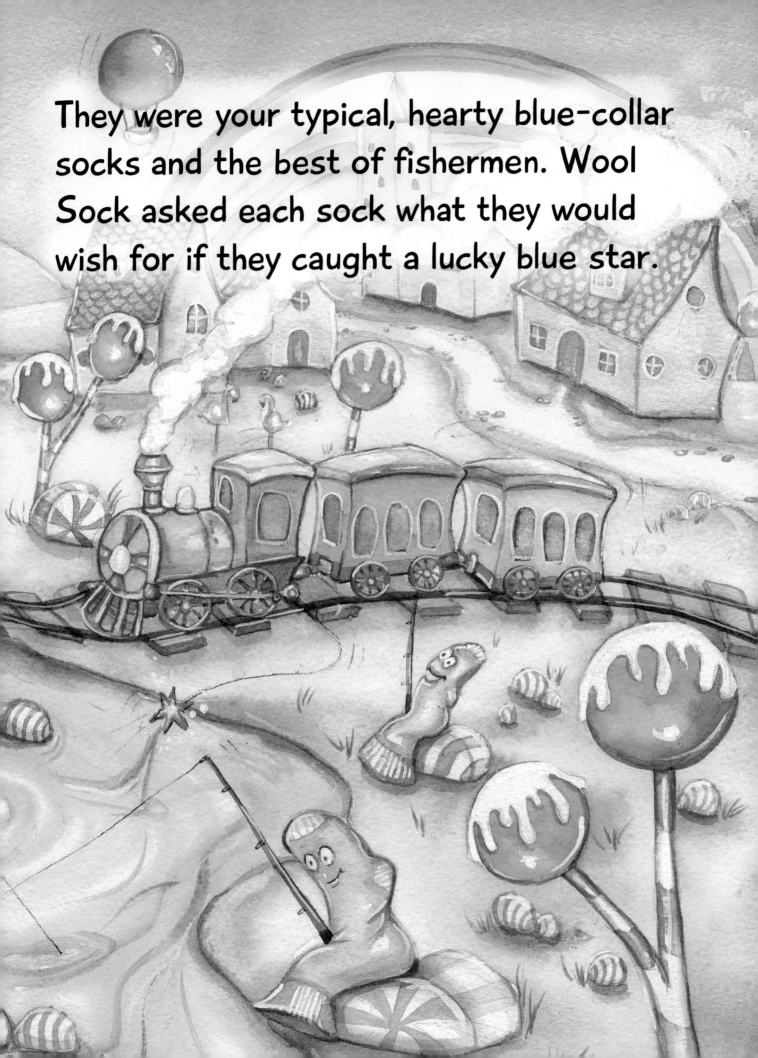

They were your typical, hearty blue-collar socks and the best of fishermen. Wool Sock asked each sock what they would wish for if they caught a lucky blue star.

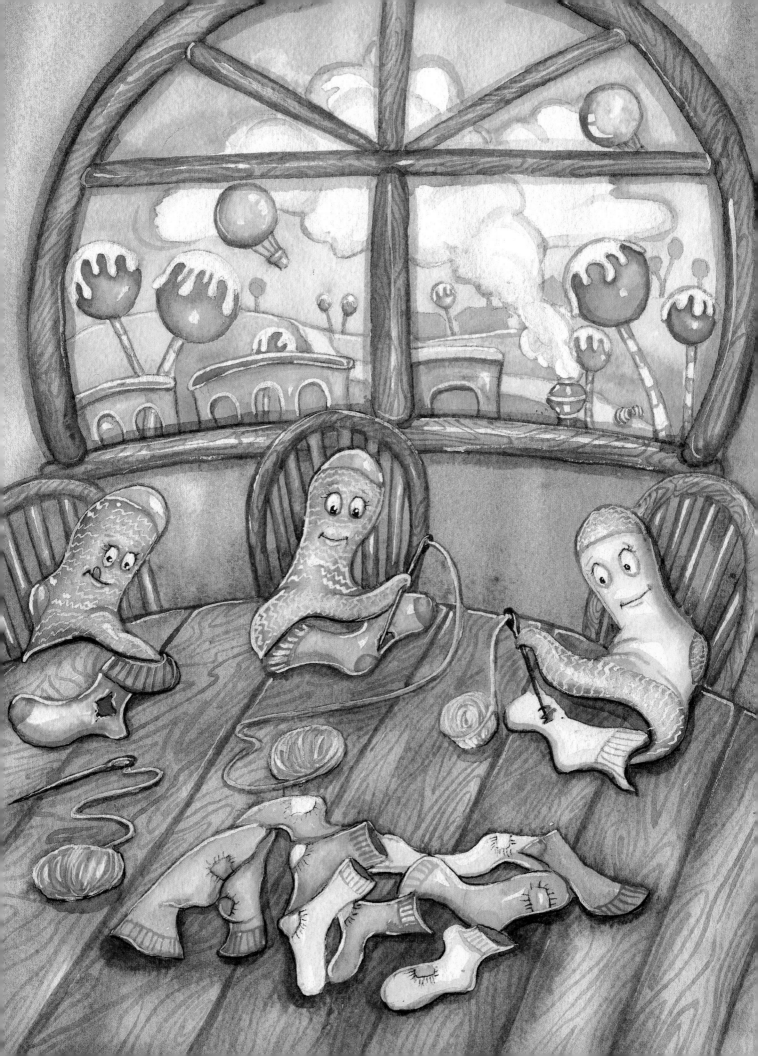

Next, the train chugged through a
neighborhood where the hand-knitted
socks lived. Those socks were made
with love and had the biggest hearts.
They usually volunteered to be caregivers
and mended the holes in other socks.
Wool Sock used that opportunity to
have each sock says something
nice about the sock
next to them.

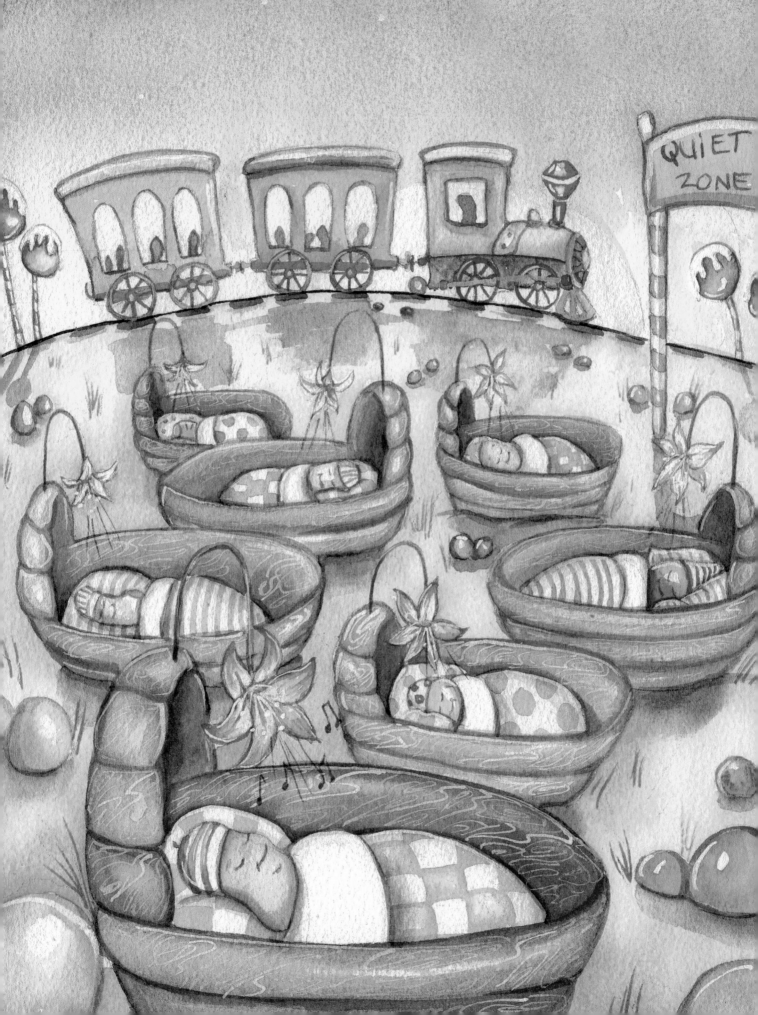

The train slowed down and refrained from blowing its whistle as it entered the quiet zone where all of the baby socks were napping. The lilies played soft lullabies, lulling them to sleep, while a timely wind tenderly rocked their cradles.

Next, the train took them through the trendiest part of town where all of the themed socks settled. It was by far the most fashionable-neighborhood to live in. Those socks were the most artistic and talented.

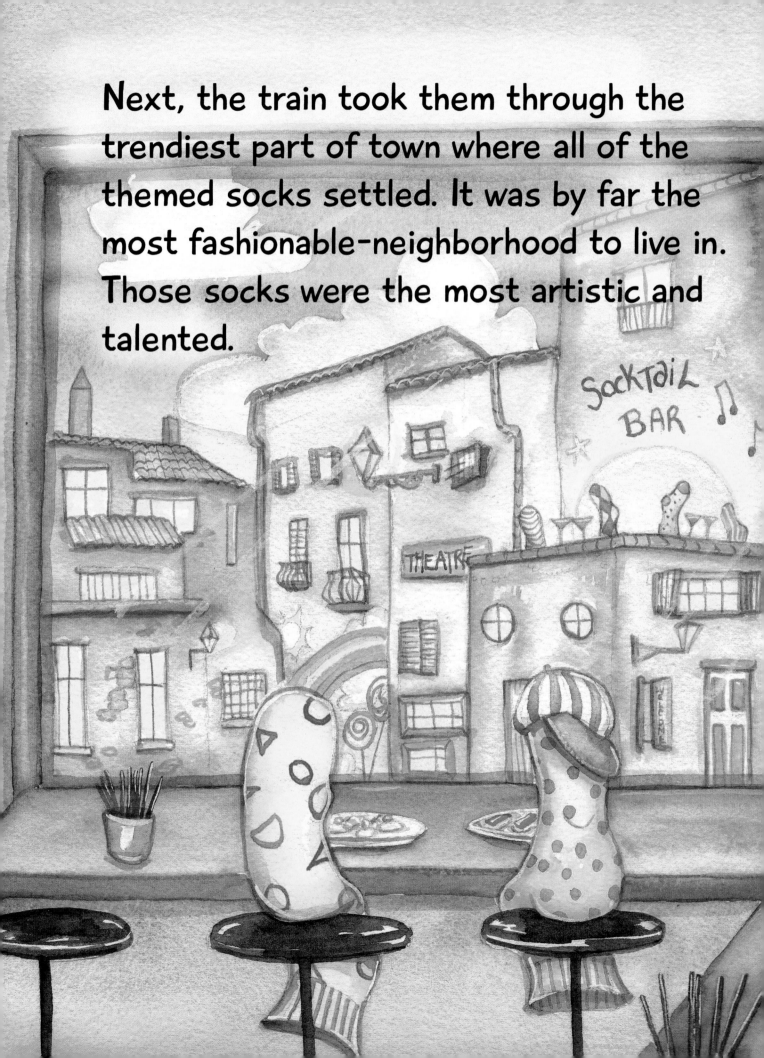

They painted pictures and murals outside of buildings and houses that reflected their favorite hobbies or interests. The themed socks enjoyed color-changing socktails on rooftop cafes and dined on candy sushi.

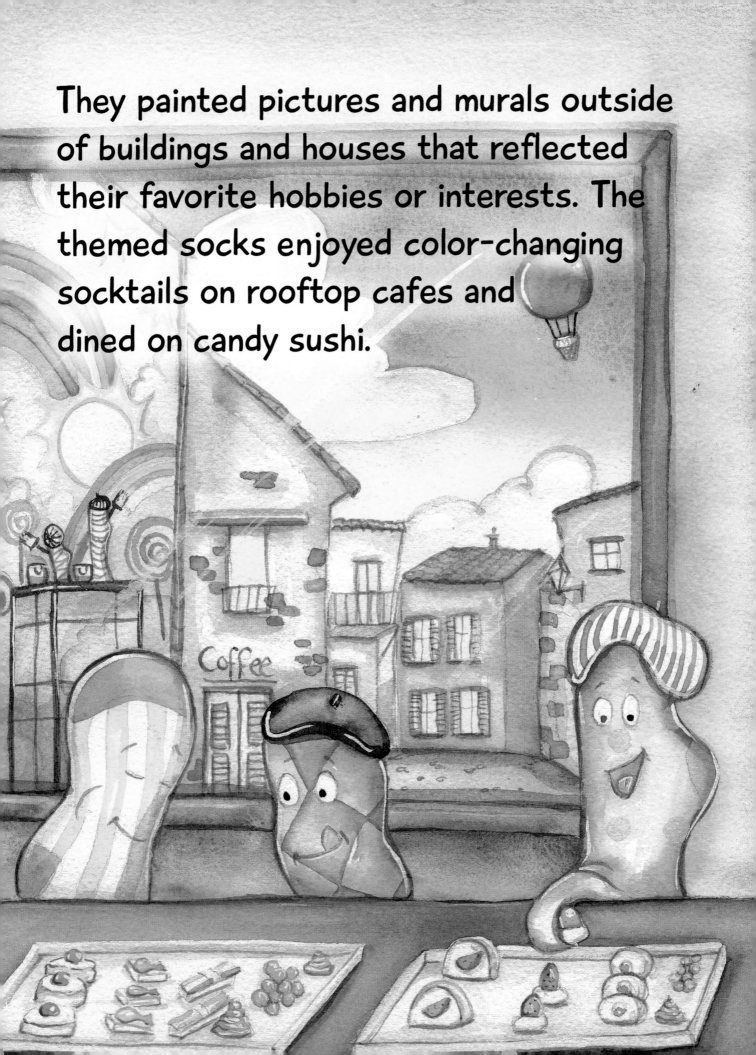

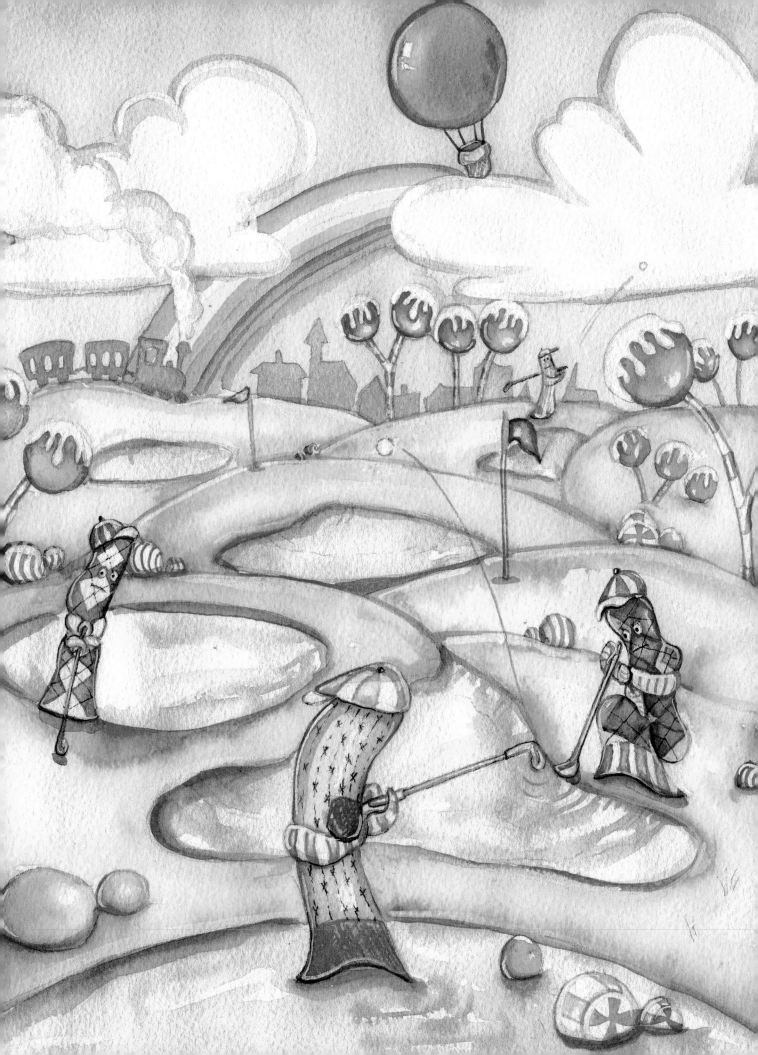

The train twisted through the part
of town where all of the silk, cashmere,
and designer socks settled.
Those socks lived a life of luxury and
spent the majority of their
time golfing. As the train
passed through, Wool
Sock asked the
socks to tell
what their
favorite hobby was.

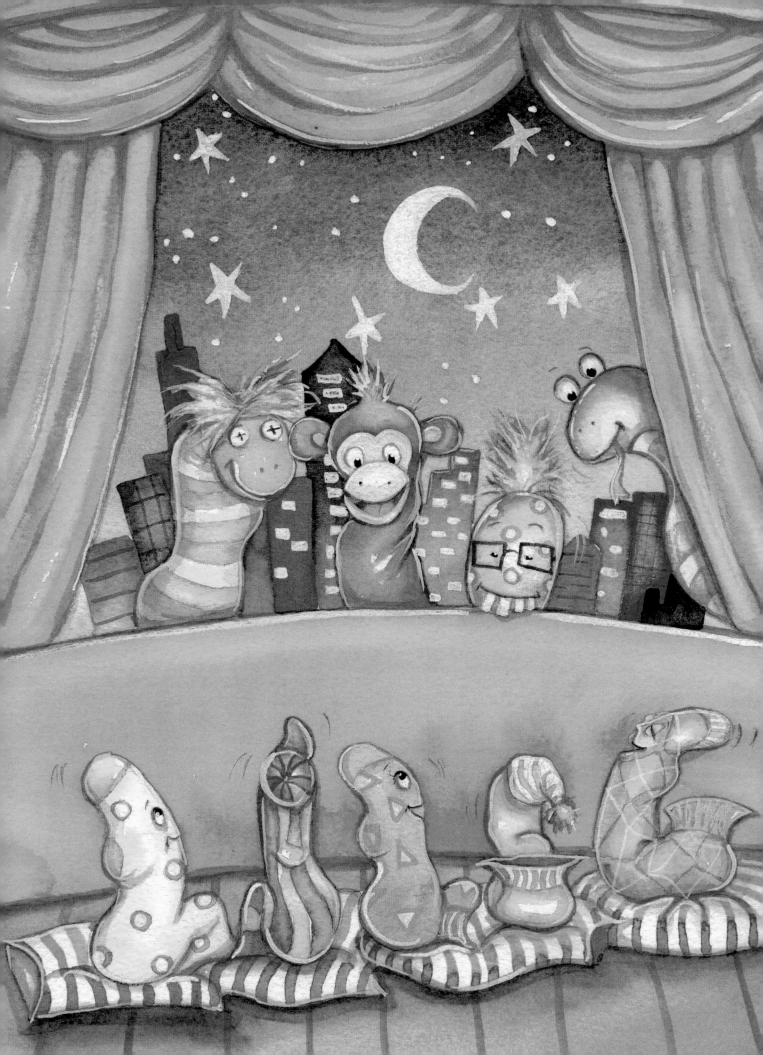

The socks that were out of style loved to reinvent themselves. Some were recycled into sock puppets or sock monkeys so they could entertain children. Many of the other unfashionable socks repurposed themselves into dusting or cleaning cloths.

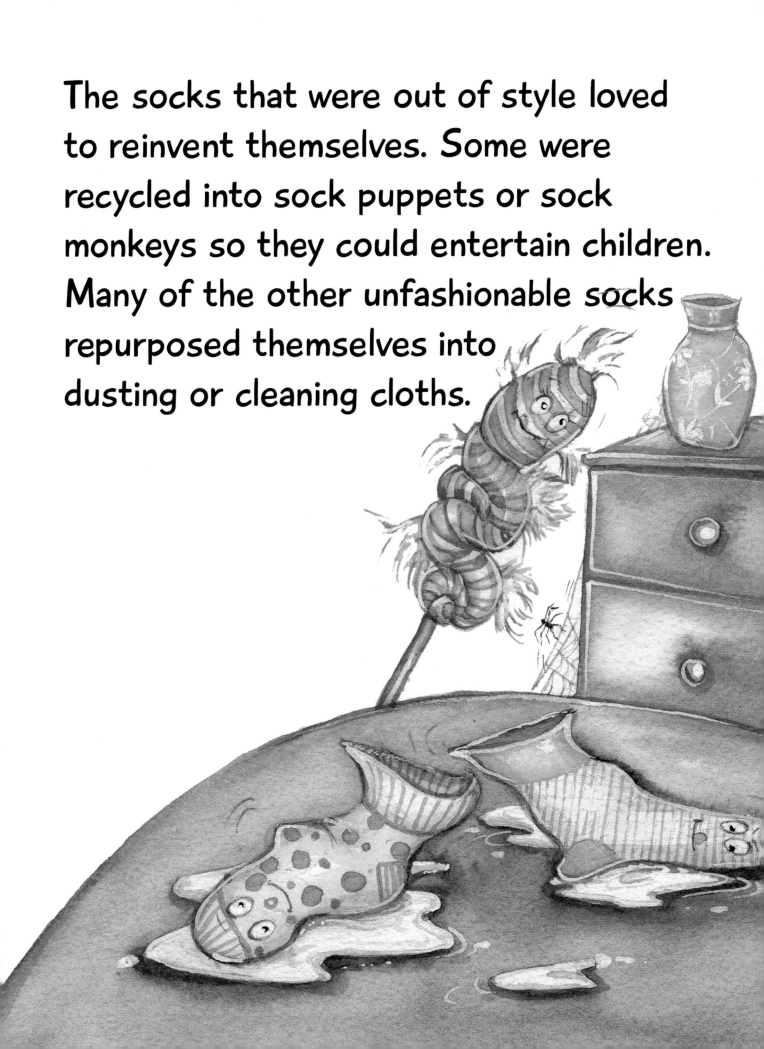

The crew socks were busy planting miniature marshmallows along the sidewalks and took turns shoveling blue pop rocks into garden beds. Some of them were diligently paving the streets with hard rock candy.

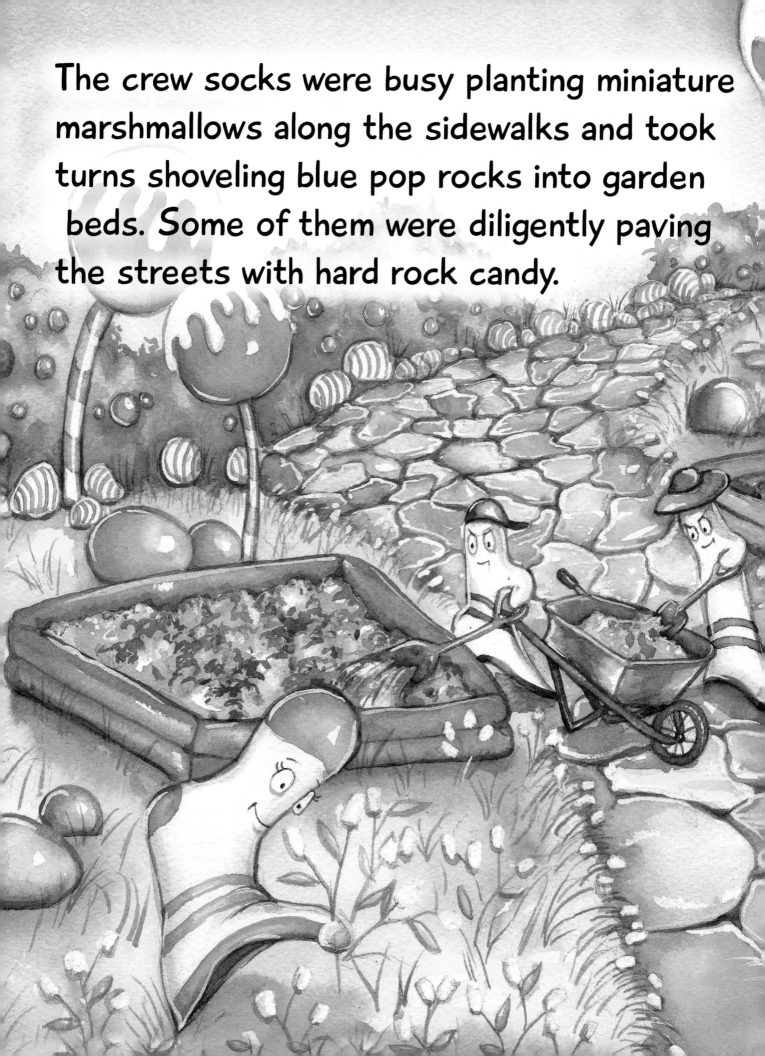

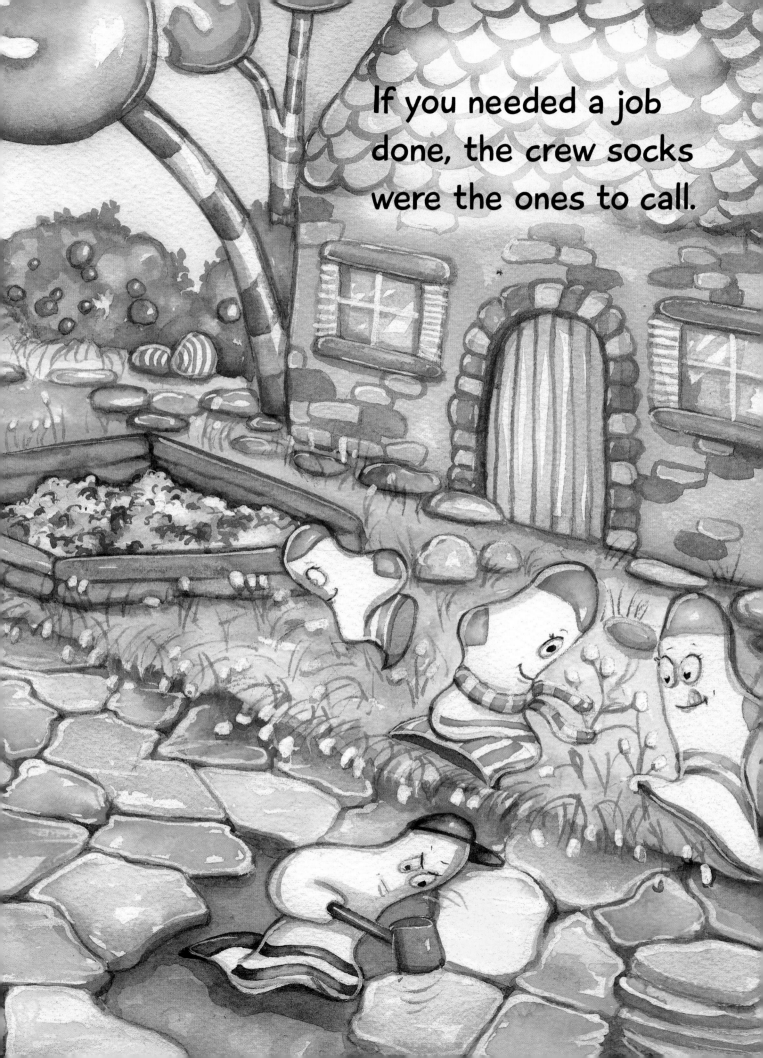

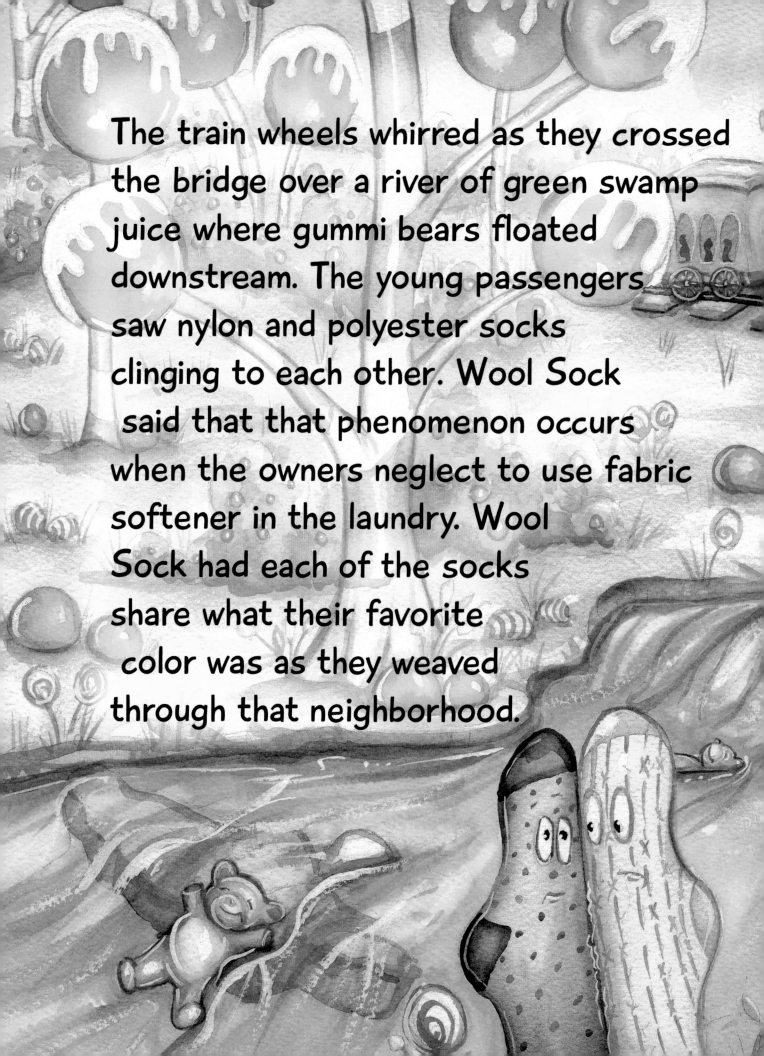

The train wheels whirred as they crossed the bridge over a river of green swamp juice where gummi bears floated downstream. The young passengers saw nylon and polyester socks clinging to each other. Wool Sock said that that phenomenon occurs when the owners neglect to use fabric softener in the laundry. Wool Sock had each of the socks share what their favorite color was as they weaved through that neighborhood.

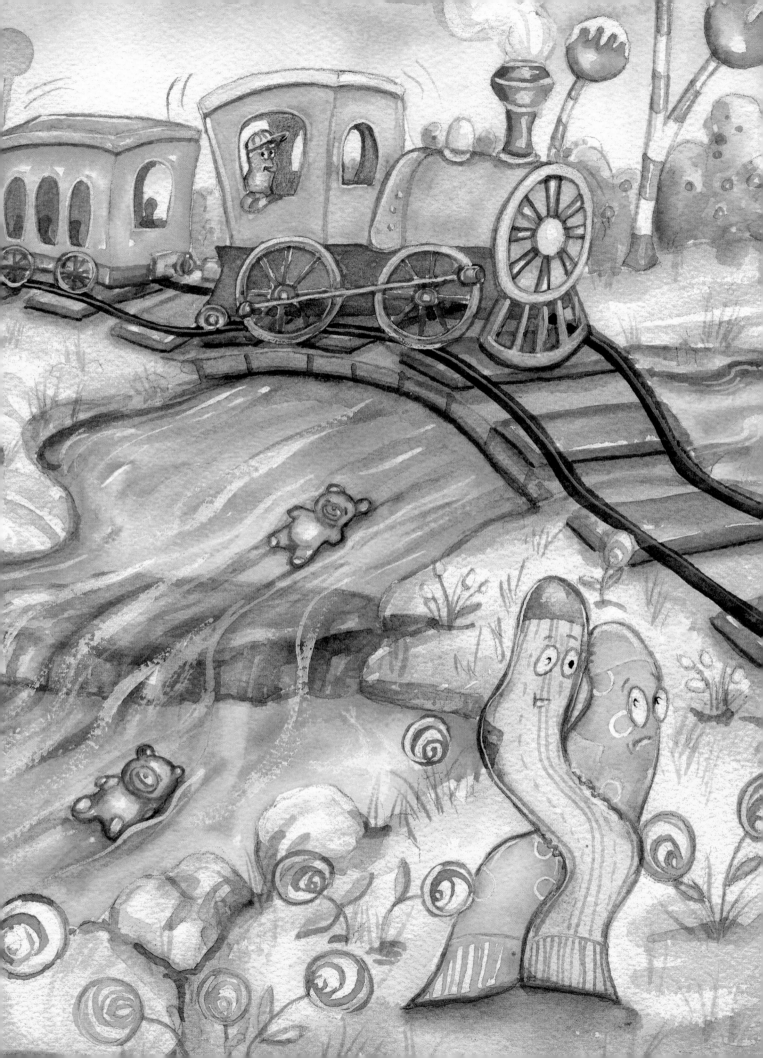

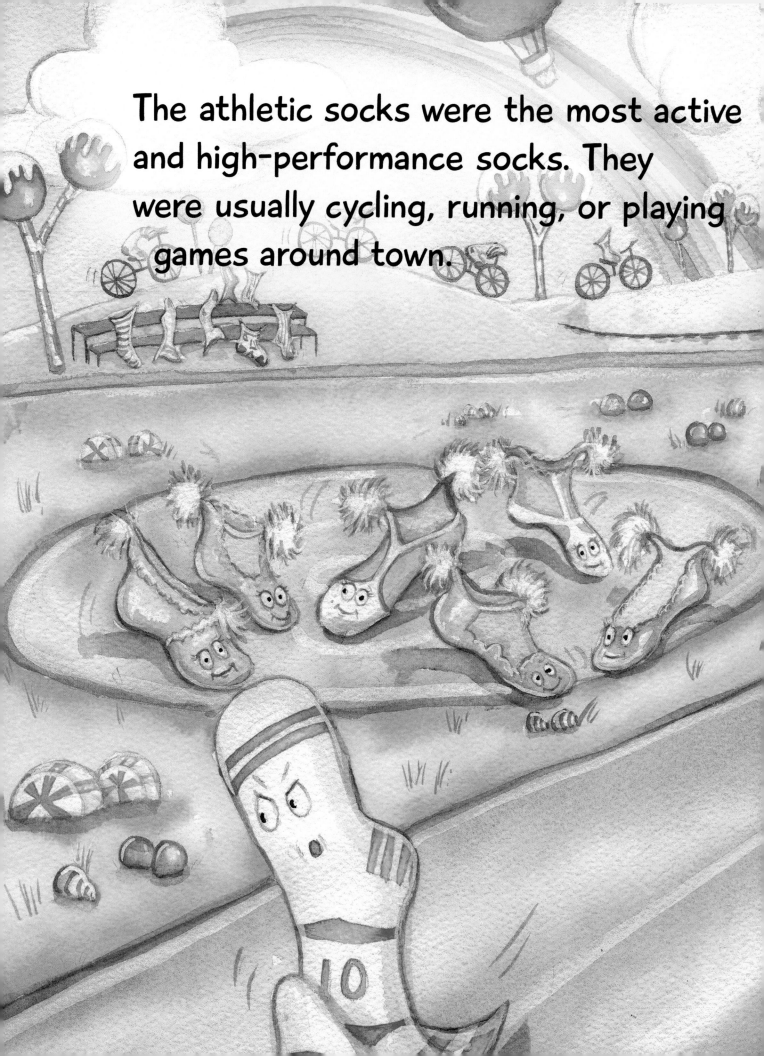

The athletic socks were the most active and high-performance socks. They were usually cycling, running, or playing games around town.

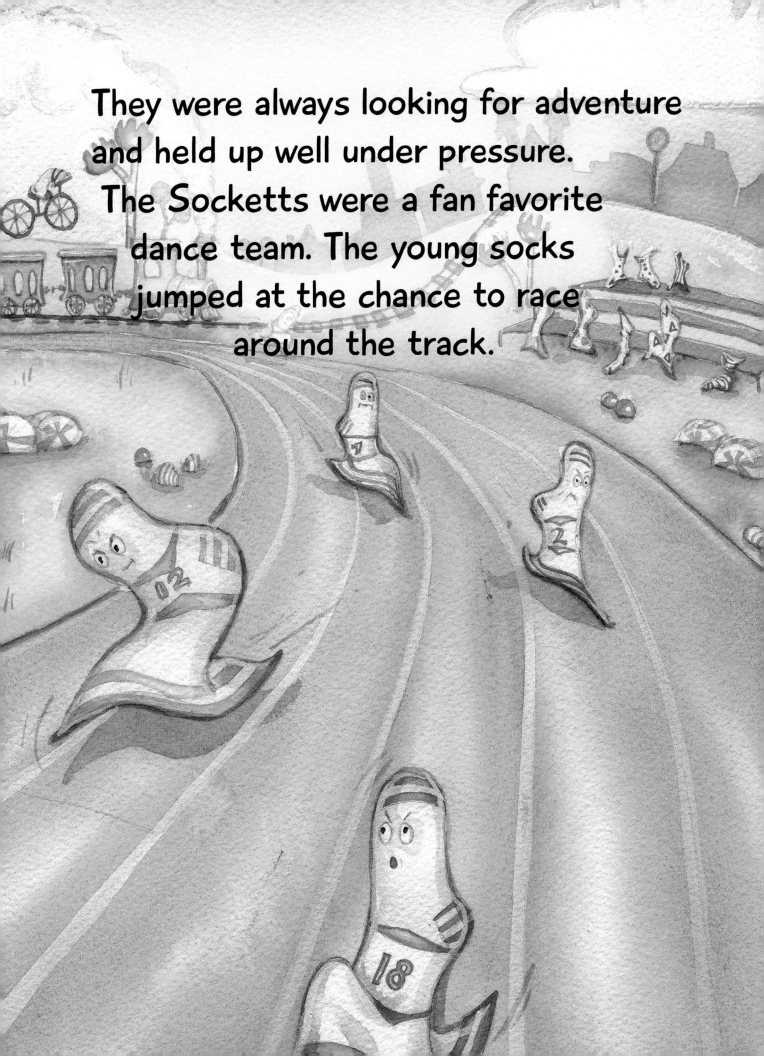

They were always looking for adventure and held up well under pressure. The Socketts were a fan favorite dance team. The young socks jumped at the chance to race around the track.

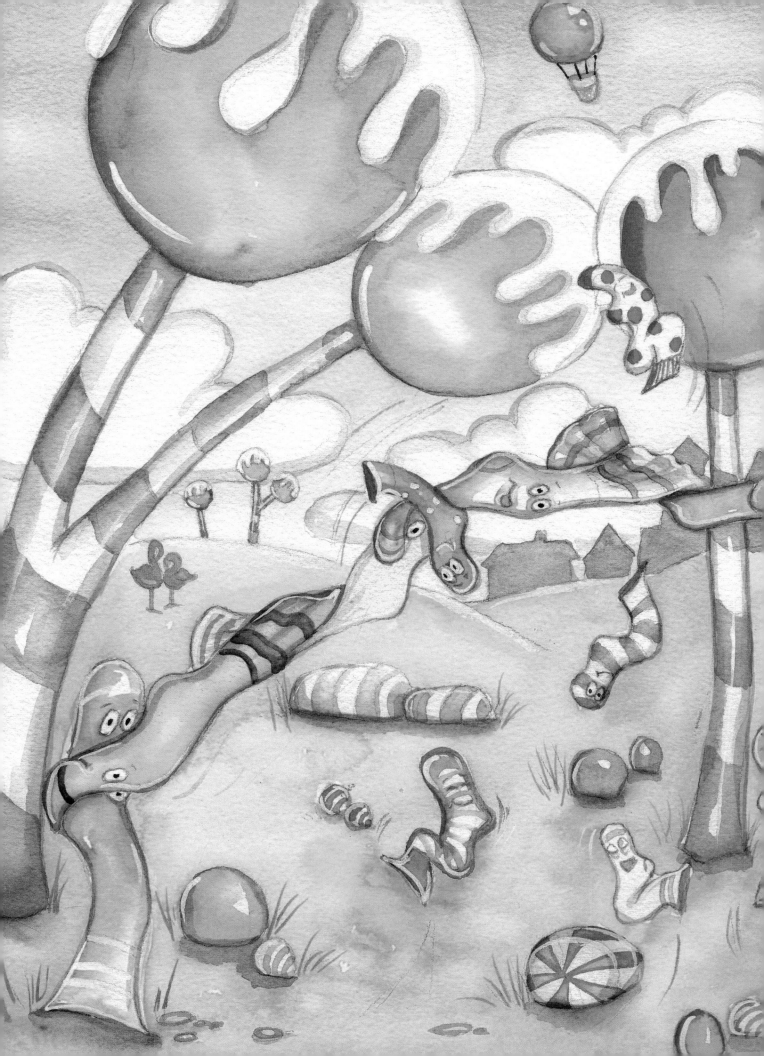

The tube socks liked to tie their ends together to make jump ropes for the younger socks. The non-slip socks were the most practical and made a career out of safety training.

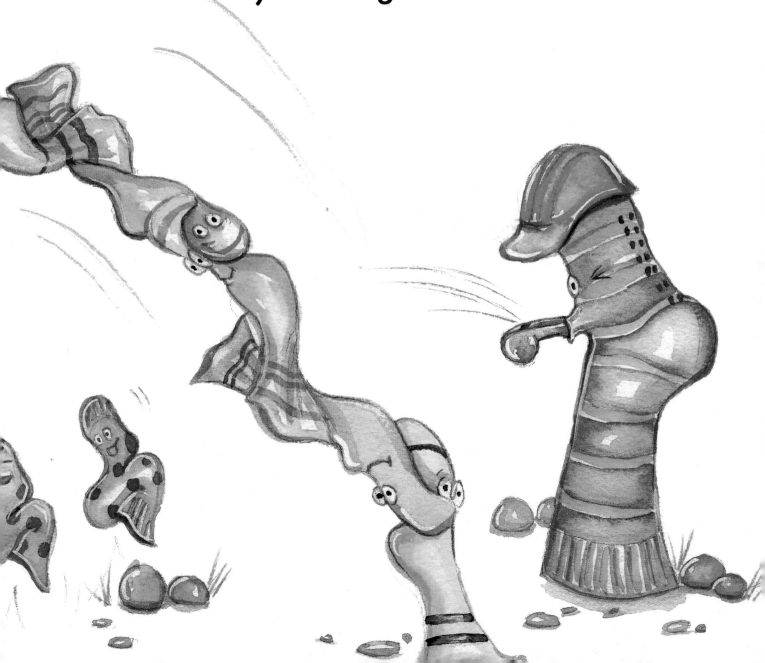

The seasonal socks took turns
decorating the whimsical little town,
and the pastry chef-inspired socks
worked in the bakeshop.
They made delicious
gluten-free cupcakes
and thumbprint cookies.
The socks sampled the
tasty treats while they
told each other what
their favorite food was.

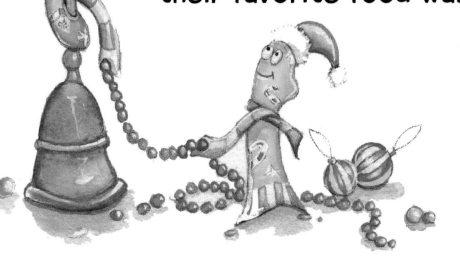

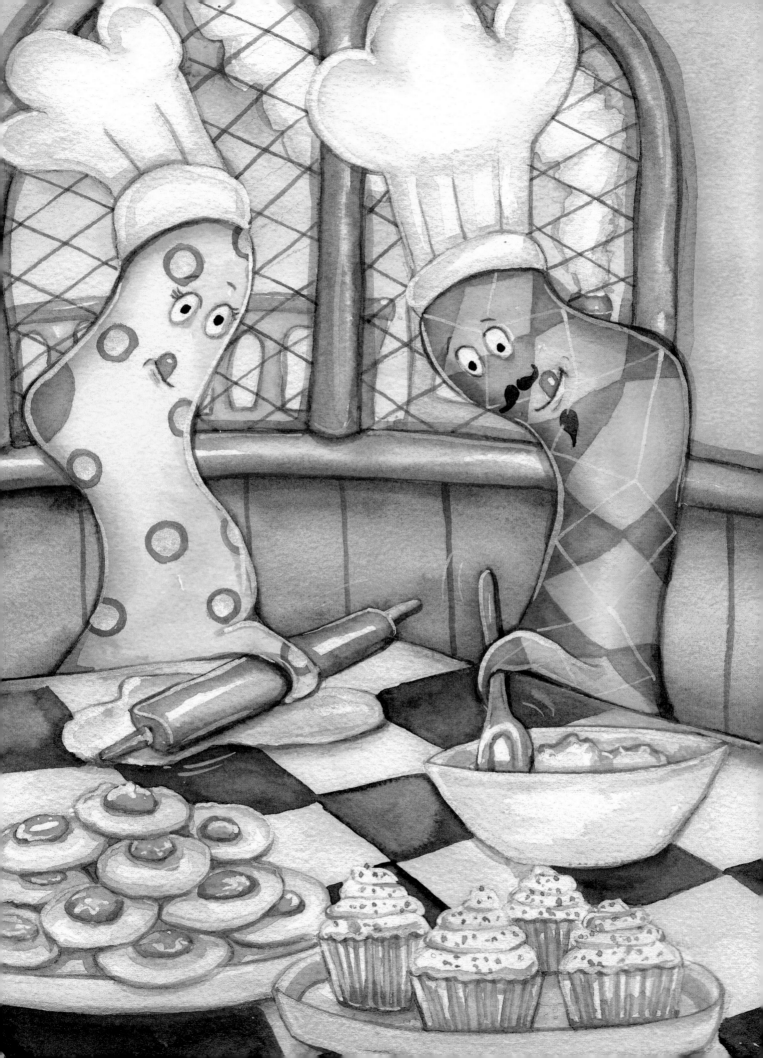

The glow-in-the-dark socks had late-night jobs. They were used in lanterns and functioned as streetlights on the corners. The yellow emoticon socks were the most popular

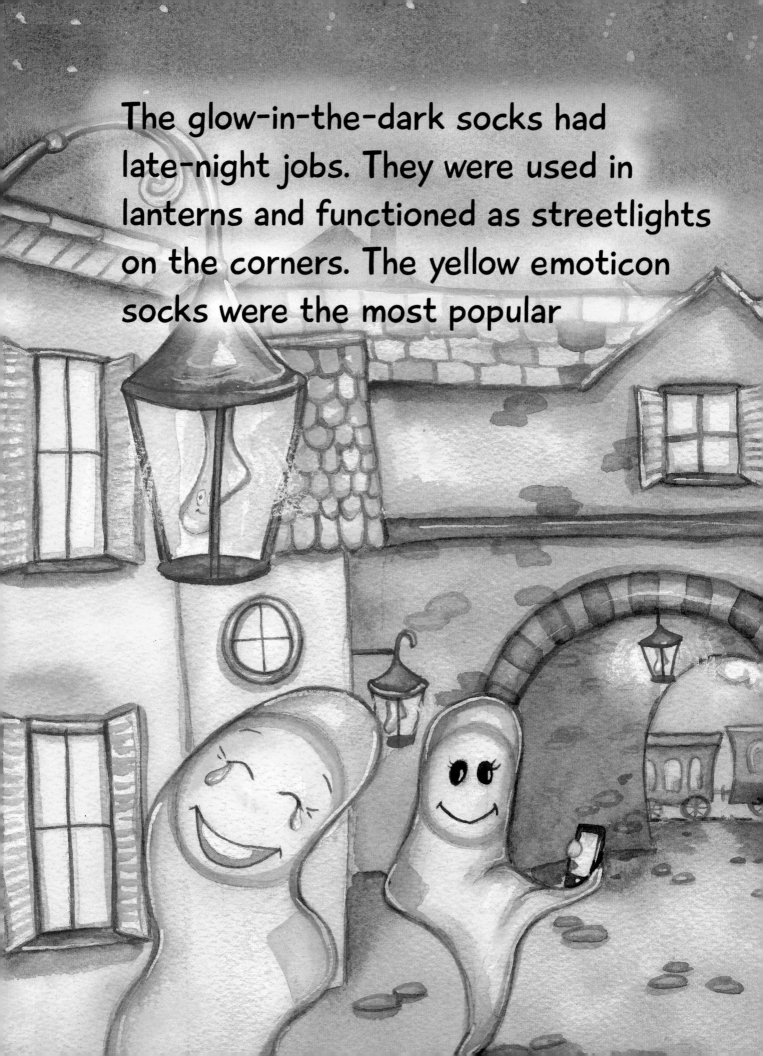

and influential socks of all time.
They had thousands of followers.
Wool Sock's strategy worked like a charm.
By the end of the day, the new socks were
talking and laughing with each other.

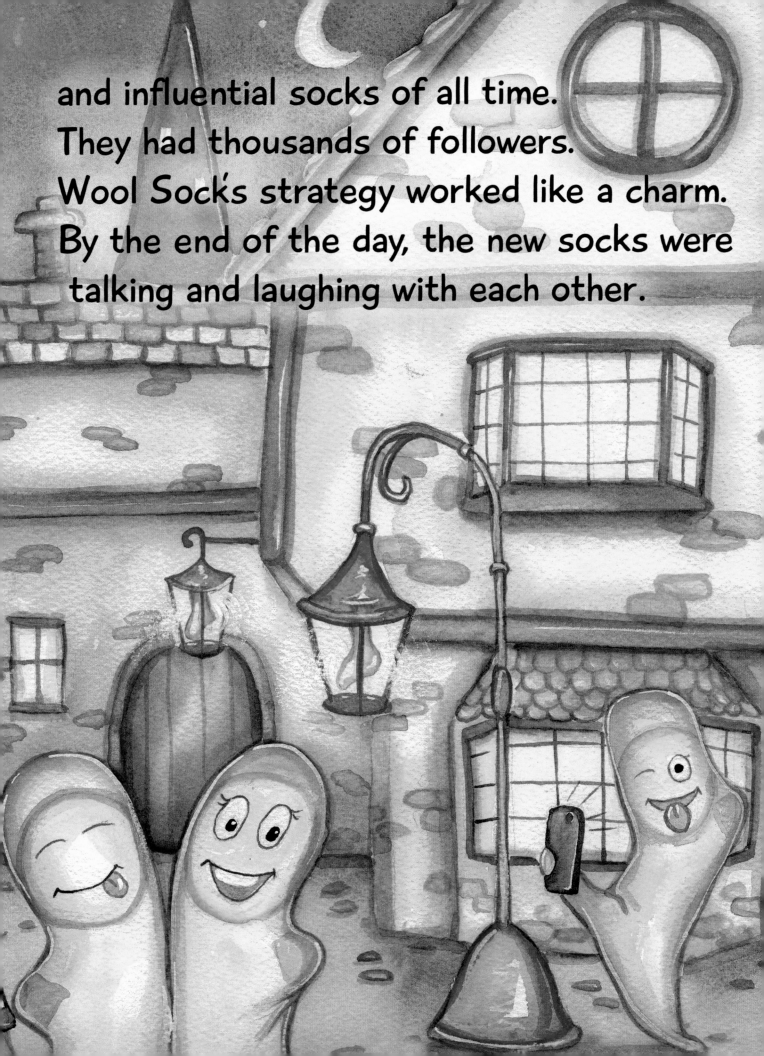

It was approaching twilight, and the passengers could see the Wishing Tree glowing in the distance.
As they got closer, they noticed that the tree had feathers on it instead of leaves, and it was twinkling from top to bottom with luminescent fireflies.

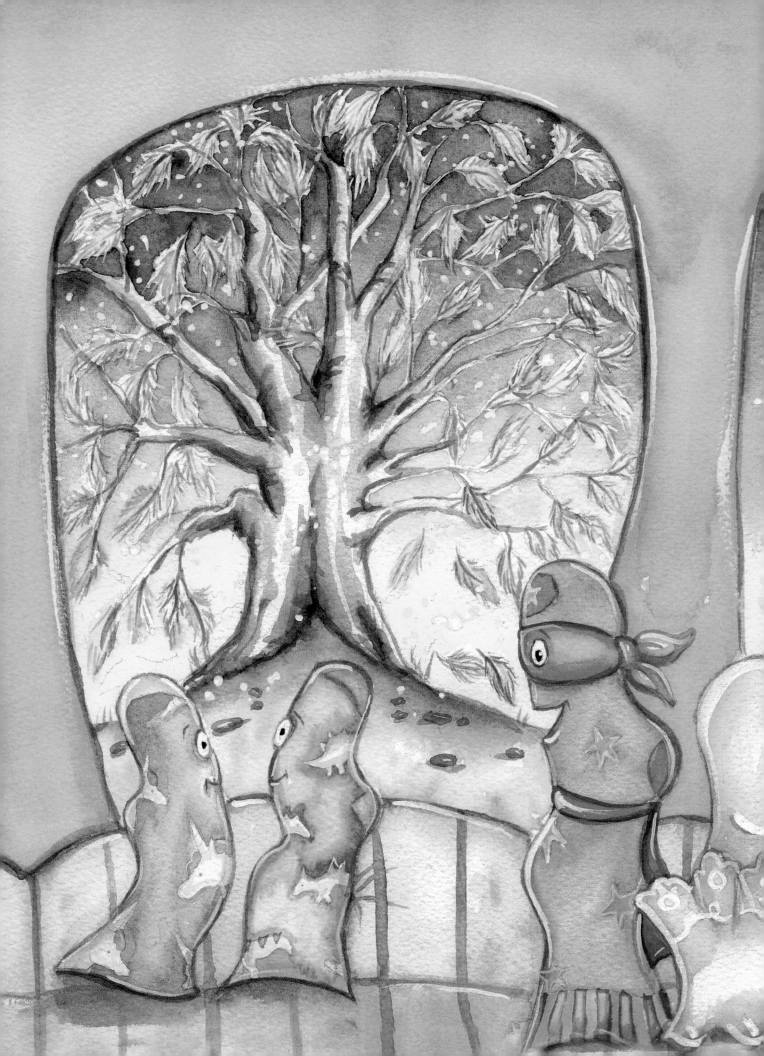

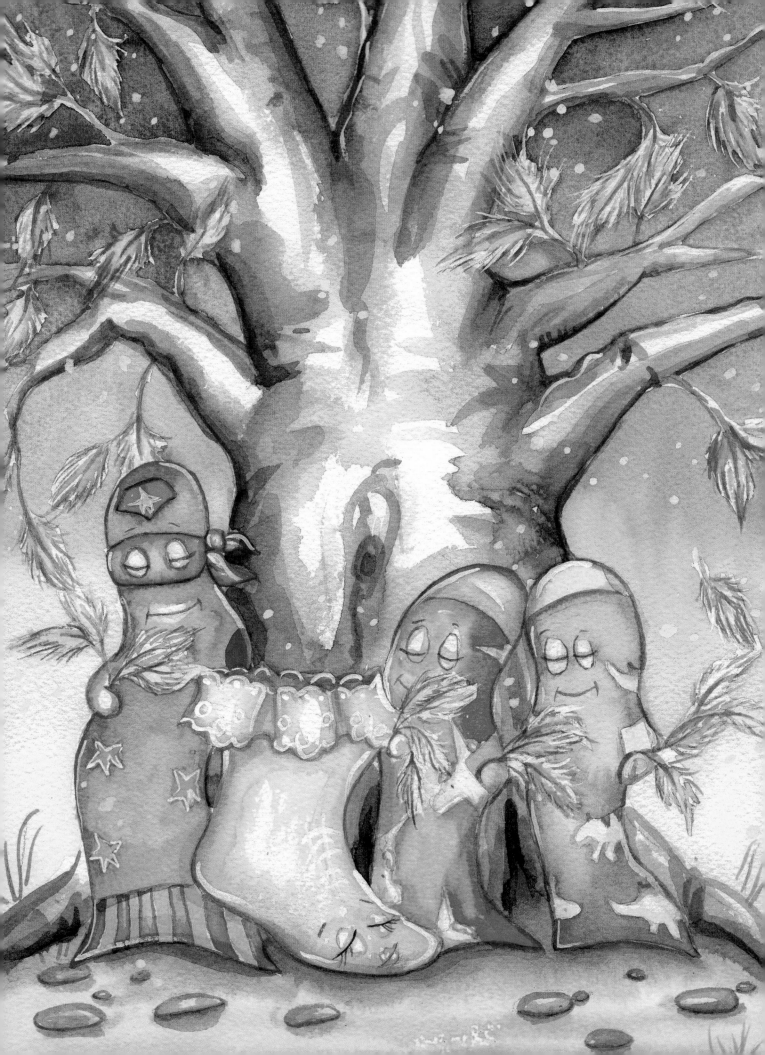

Wool Sock instructed the passenger socks to take a place under the Wishing Tree. They were each given a cluster of magical feathers and were told to close their eyes and make a wish to stay or go back home.

When they opened their eyes, all four socks were still there. They all wished to stay.

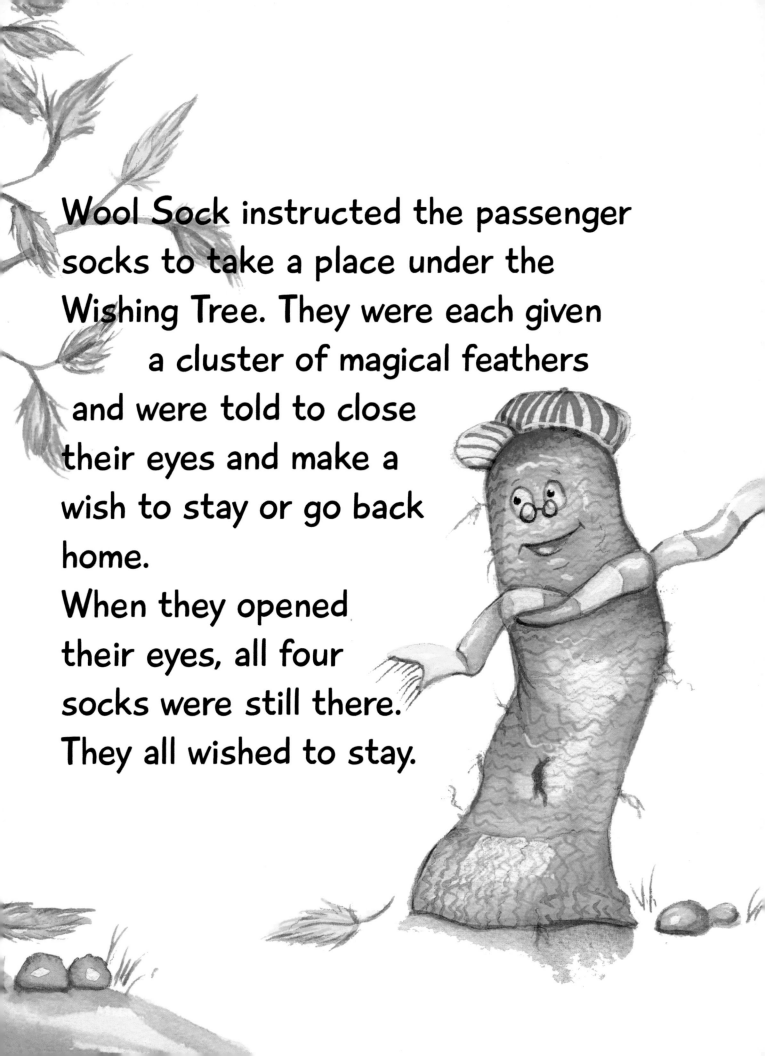

Change can be scary,
but friendships were
made on the train that
   day. It made the transition
   much smoother. They loved what
   they saw of the town and their new
friends. Sometimes things fall apart so
something better can fall together.
It was the best thing that happened
   to the new socks. Pendrell, Pink Ankle
Sock, Dinosaur, and Unicorn Sock now
live inside a cozy fairytale where there
is no better place to be.
What kind of sock would you be?


The End

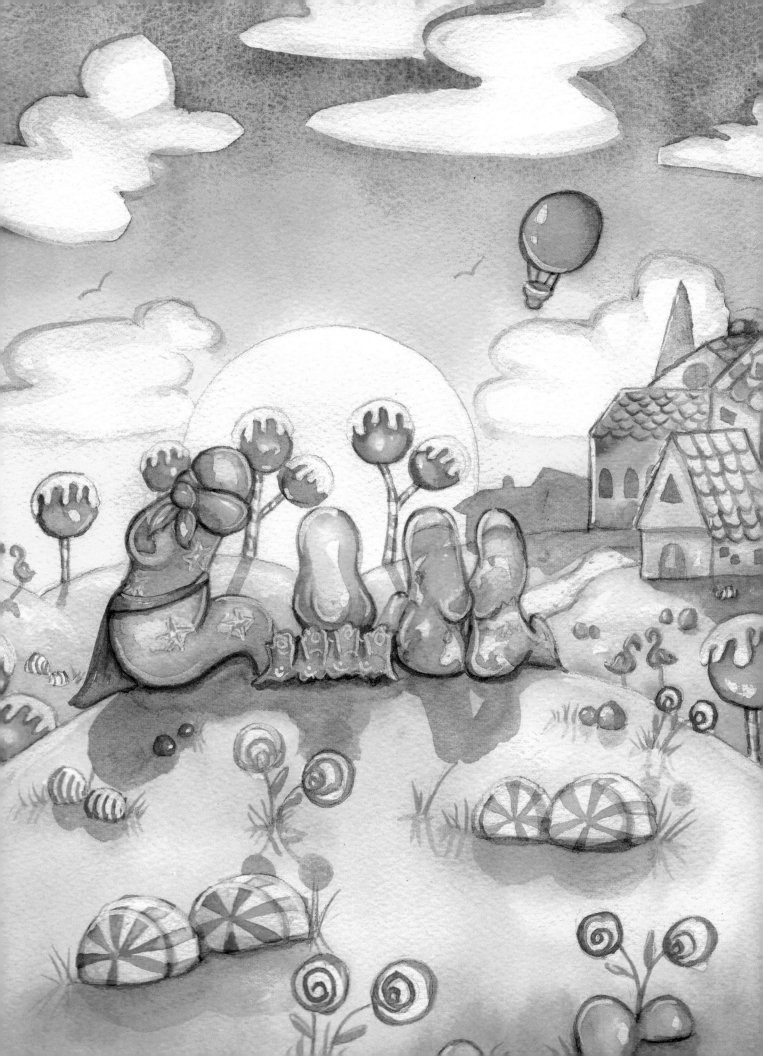

Made in the USA
Middletown, DE
08 February 2024

49358397R00031